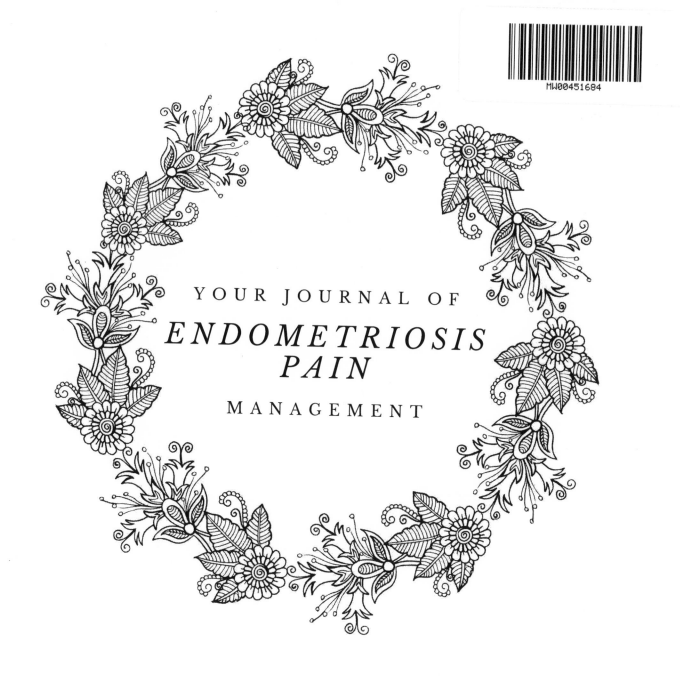

YOUR JOURNAL OF

ENDOMETRIOSIS PAIN

MANAGEMENT

Use this journal to track your pain levels, moods, meditations, medications, self-care and more.

Journal your thoughts and track achievements.

Throughout this book there are inspirational quotes to direct you away from negative feelings of guilt and depression. There are also journal prompts and CBT inspired exercise pages to find more productive patterns of behaviour.

There are affirmation pages, gratitude pages, trigger tracking pages and more.

You are not alone - wishing you luck and love.

WEEKLY MOOD & PAIN TRACKER - PLOT YOUR MOOD AND PAIN ON THE GRAPH IN DIFFERENT COLORS, KEEP NOTE OF YOUR TRIGGERS BELOW.

PAIN LEVEL

0
1
2
3
4
5
6
7
8
9
10
11
12
13
14
15
16
17

MONDAY	TUESDAY	WEDNESDAY	THURSDAY	FRIDAY	SATURDAY	SUNDAY

TIME OF DAY PAIN TRACKER ⏱

MORNING

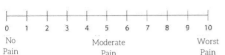

0 1 2 3 4 5 6 7 8 9 10
No Pain   Moderate Pain   Worst Pain

AFTERNOON

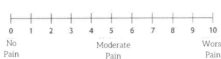

0 1 2 3 4 5 6 7 8 9 10
No Pain   Moderate Pain   Worst Pain

EVENING

0 1 2 3 4 5 6 7 8 9 10
No Pain   Moderate Pain   Worst Pain

MORNING

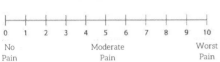

0 1 2 3 4 5 6 7 8 9 10
No Pain   Moderate Pain   Worst Pain

AFTERNOON

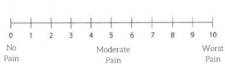

0 1 2 3 4 5 6 7 8 9 10
No Pain   Moderate Pain   Worst Pain

EVENING

0 1 2 3 4 5 6 7 8 9 10
No Pain   Moderate Pain   Worst Pain

MORNING

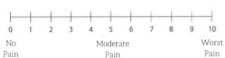

0 1 2 3 4 5 6 7 8 9 10
No Pain   Moderate Pain   Worst Pain

AFTERNOON

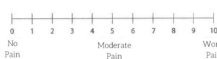

0 1 2 3 4 5 6 7 8 9 10
No Pain   Moderate Pain   Worst Pain

EVENING

0 1 2 3 4 5 6 7 8 9 10
No Pain   Moderate Pain   Worst Pain

MORNING

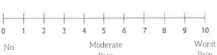

0 1 2 3 4 5 6 7 8 9 10
No Pain   Moderate Pain   Worst Pain

AFTERNOON

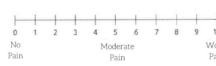

0 1 2 3 4 5 6 7 8 9 10
No Pain   Moderate Pain   Worst Pain

EVENING

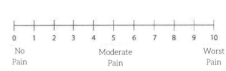

0 1 2 3 4 5 6 7 8 9 10
No Pain   Moderate Pain   Worst Pain

MORNING

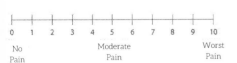

0 1 2 3 4 5 6 7 8 9 10
No Pain   Moderate Pain   Worst Pain

AFTERNOON

0 1 2 3 4 5 6 7 8 9 10
No Pain   Moderate Pain   Worst Pain

EVENING

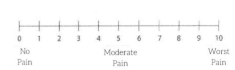

0 1 2 3 4 5 6 7 8 9 10
No Pain   Moderate Pain   Worst Pain

WHAT DOES GRATITUDE MEAN?

ANSWER THESE QUESTIONS TO BREAK OUT OF NEGATIVE THOUGHT PATTERNS AND REFOCUS ON THE THINGS THAT MAKE YOU HAPPY AND GRATEFUL.

_____
_____
_____
_____
_____
_____
_____
_____
_____
_____
_____
_____
_____
_____
_____
_____
_____
_____
_____
_____
_____
_____
_____

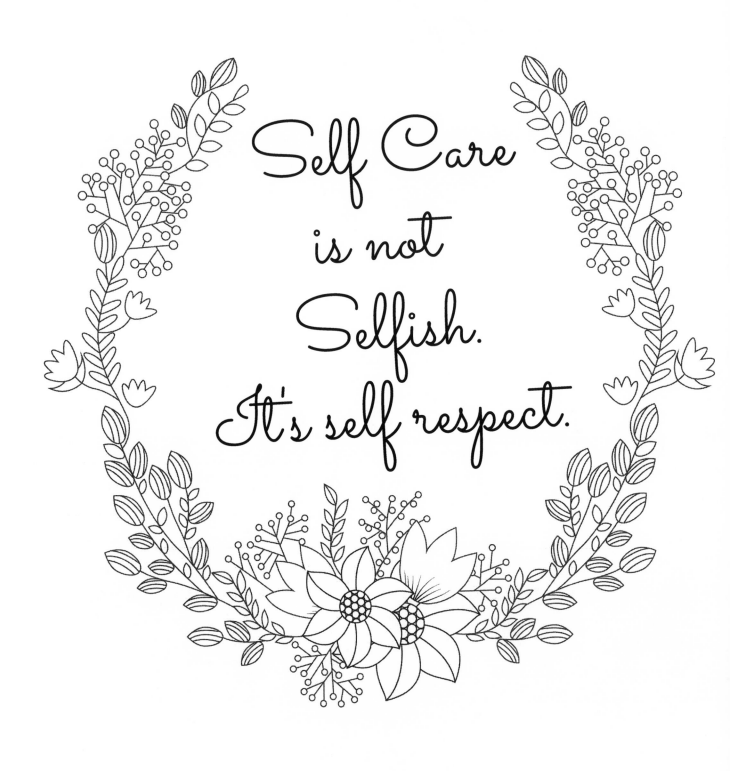

WEEKLY MOOD & PAIN TRACKER - PLOT YOUR MOOD AND PAIN ON THE GRAPH IN DIFFERENT COLORS, KEEP NOTE OF YOUR TRIGGERS BELOW.

PAIN LEVEL

0
1
2
3
4
5
6
7
8
9
10
11
12
13
14
15
16
17

| MONDAY | TUESDAY | WEDNESDAY | THURSDAY | FRIDAY | SATURDAY | SUNDAY |

TIME OF DAY PAIN TRACKER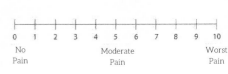

MORNING

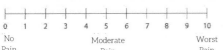

0 1 2 3 4 5 6 7 8 9 10
No Pain   Moderate Pain   Worst Pain

AFTERNOON

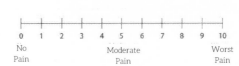

0 1 2 3 4 5 6 7 8 9 10
No Pain   Moderate Pain   Worst Pain

EVENING

0 1 2 3 4 5 6 7 8 9 10
No Pain   Moderate Pain   Worst Pain

MORNING

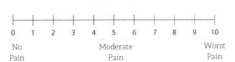

0 1 2 3 4 5 6 7 8 9 10
No Pain   Moderate Pain   Worst Pain

AFTERNOON

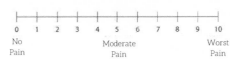

0 1 2 3 4 5 6 7 8 9 10
No Pain   Moderate Pain   Worst Pain

EVENING

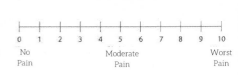

0 1 2 3 4 5 6 7 8 9 10
No Pain   Moderate Pain   Worst Pain

MORNING

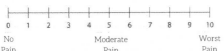

0 1 2 3 4 5 6 7 8 9 10
No Pain   Moderate Pain   Worst Pain

AFTERNOON

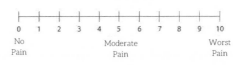

0 1 2 3 4 5 6 7 8 9 10
No Pain   Moderate Pain   Worst Pain

EVENING

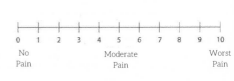

0 1 2 3 4 5 6 7 8 9 10
No Pain   Moderate Pain   Worst Pain

MORNING

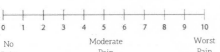

0 1 2 3 4 5 6 7 8 9 10
No Pain   Moderate Pain   Worst Pain

AFTERNOON

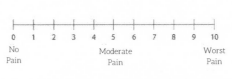

0 1 2 3 4 5 6 7 8 9 10
No Pain   Moderate Pain   Worst Pain

EVENING

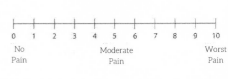

0 1 2 3 4 5 6 7 8 9 10
No Pain   Moderate Pain   Worst Pain

MORNING

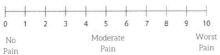

0 1 2 3 4 5 6 7 8 9 10
No Pain   Moderate Pain   Worst Pain

AFTERNOON

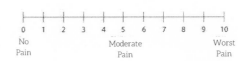

0 1 2 3 4 5 6 7 8 9 10
No Pain   Moderate Pain   Worst Pain

EVENING

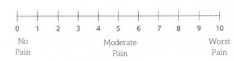

0 1 2 3 4 5 6 7 8 9 10
No Pain   Moderate Pain   Worst Pain

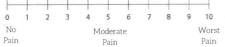
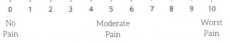
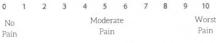
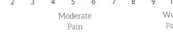

WEEKLY MOOD & PAIN TRACKER - PLOT YOUR MOOD AND PAIN ON THE GRAPH IN DIFFERENT COLORS, KEEP NOTE OF YOUR TRIGGERS BELOW.

PAIN LEVEL

0

1

2

3

4

5

6

7

8

9

10

11

12

13

14

15

16

17

MONDAY   TUESDAY   WEDNESDAY   THURSDAY   FRIDAY   SATURDAY   SUNDAY

TIME OF DAY PAIN TRACKER

MORNING
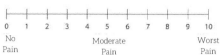

0 1 2 3 4 5 6 7 8 9 10
No Pain   Moderate Pain   Worst Pain

AFTERNOON
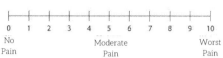

0 1 2 3 4 5 6 7 8 9 10
No Pain   Moderate Pain   Worst Pain

EVENING
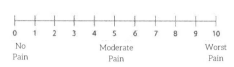

0 1 2 3 4 5 6 7 8 9 10
No Pain   Moderate Pain   Worst Pain

MORNING
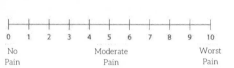

0 1 2 3 4 5 6 7 8 9 10
No Pain   Moderate Pain   Worst Pain

AFTERNOON
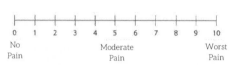

0 1 2 3 4 5 6 7 8 9 10
No Pain   Moderate Pain   Worst Pain

EVENING
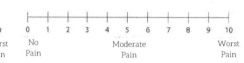

0 1 2 3 4 5 6 7 8 9 10
No Pain   Moderate Pain   Worst Pain

MORNING
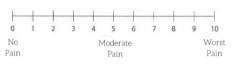

0 1 2 3 4 5 6 7 8 9 10
No Pain   Moderate Pain   Worst Pain

AFTERNOON
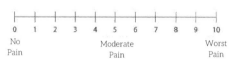

0 1 2 3 4 5 6 7 8 9 10
No Pain   Moderate Pain   Worst Pain

EVENING
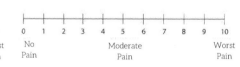

0 1 2 3 4 5 6 7 8 9 10
No Pain   Moderate Pain   Worst Pain

MORNING
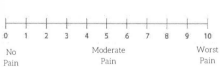

0 1 2 3 4 5 6 7 8 9 10
No Pain   Moderate Pain   Worst Pain

AFTERNOON
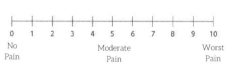

0 1 2 3 4 5 6 7 8 9 10
No Pain   Moderate Pain   Worst Pain

EVENING
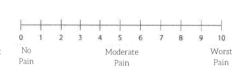

0 1 2 3 4 5 6 7 8 9 10
No Pain   Moderate Pain   Worst Pain

MORNING
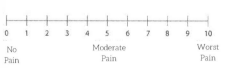

0 1 2 3 4 5 6 7 8 9 10
No Pain   Moderate Pain   Worst Pain

AFTERNOON
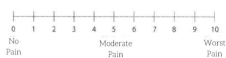

0 1 2 3 4 5 6 7 8 9 10
No Pain   Moderate Pain   Worst Pain

EVENING
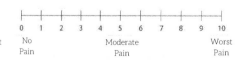

0 1 2 3 4 5 6 7 8 9 10
No Pain   Moderate Pain   Worst Pain

WHEN IS IT IMPORTANT TO BE GRATEFUL?

ANSWER THESE QUESTIONS TO BREAK OUT OF NEGATIVE
THOUGHT PATTERNS AND REFOCUS ON THE THINGS THAT MAKE
YOU HAPPY AND GRATEFUL.

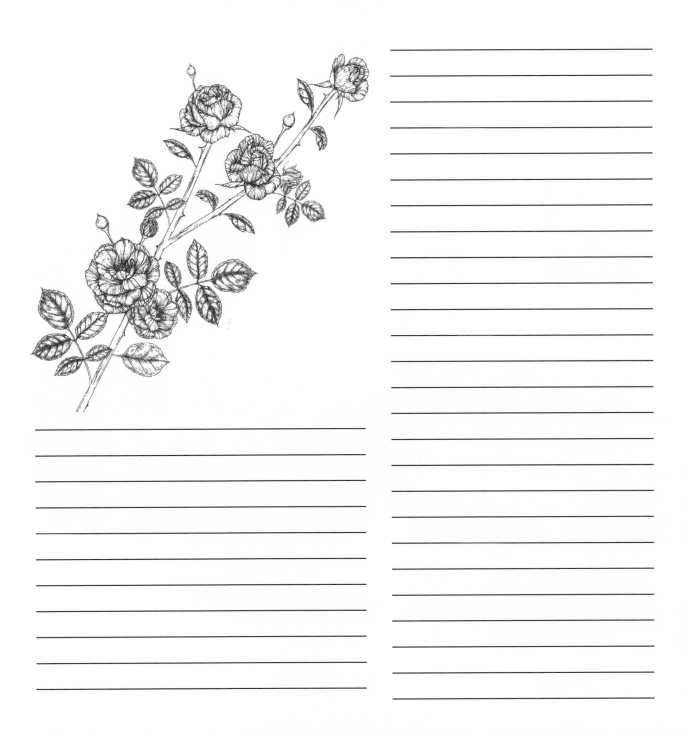

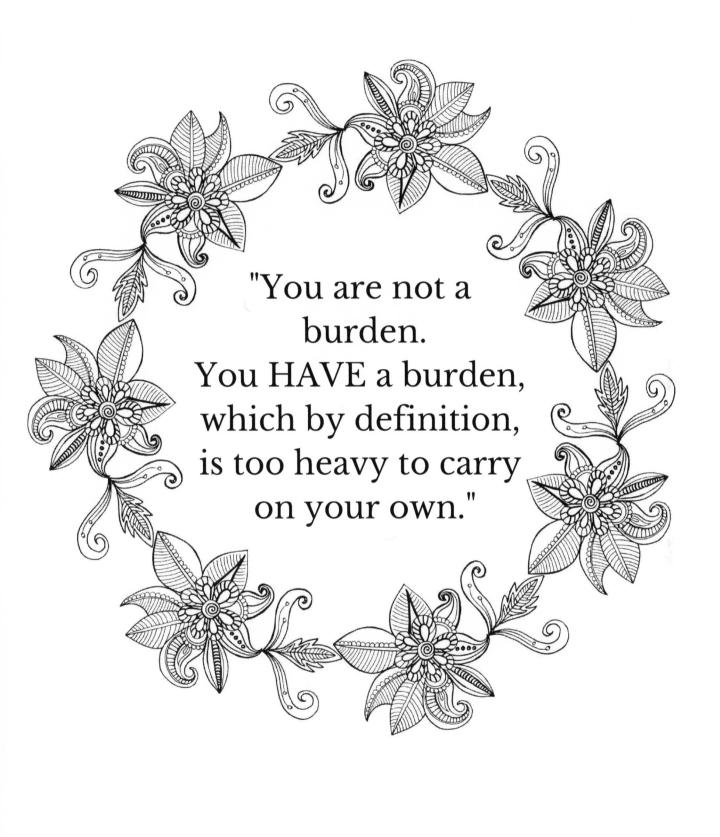

"You are not a
burden.
You HAVE a burden,
which by definition,
is too heavy to carry
on your own."

WEEKLY MOOD & PAIN TRACKER - PLOT YOUR MOOD AND PAIN ON THE GRAPH IN DIFFERENT COLORS, KEEP NOTE OF YOUR TRIGGERS BELOW.

PAIN LEVEL

0
1
2
3
4
5
6
7
8
9
10
11
12
13
14
15
16
17

MONDAY   TUESDAY   WEDNESDAY   THURSDAY   FRIDAY   SATURDAY   SUNDAY

TIME OF DAY PAIN TRACKER

MORNING
0 1 2 3 4 5 6 7 8 9 10
No Pain   Moderate Pain   Worst Pain

AFTERNOON
0 1 2 3 4 5 6 7 8 9 10
No Pain   Moderate Pain   Worst Pain

EVENING
0 1 2 3 4 5 6 7 8 9 10
No Pain   Moderate Pain   Worst Pain

MORNING
0 1 2 3 4 5 6 7 8 9 10
No Pain   Moderate Pain   Worst Pain

AFTERNOON
0 1 2 3 4 5 6 7 8 9 10
No Pain   Moderate Pain   Worst Pain

EVENING
0 1 2 3 4 5 6 7 8 9 10
No Pain   Moderate Pain   Worst Pain

MORNING
0 1 2 3 4 5 6 7 8 9 10
No Pain   Moderate Pain   Worst Pain

AFTERNOON
0 1 2 3 4 5 6 7 8 9 10
No Pain   Moderate Pain   Worst Pain

EVENING
0 1 2 3 4 5 6 7 8 9 10
No Pain   Moderate Pain   Worst Pain

MORNING
0 1 2 3 4 5 6 7 8 9 10
No Pain   Moderate Pain   Worst Pain

AFTERNOON
0 1 2 3 4 5 6 7 8 9 10
No Pain   Moderate Pain   Worst Pain

EVENING
0 1 2 3 4 5 6 7 8 9 10
No Pain   Moderate Pain   Worst Pain

MORNING
0 1 2 3 4 5 6 7 8 9 10
No Pain   Moderate Pain   Worst Pain

AFTERNOON
0 1 2 3 4 5 6 7 8 9 10
No Pain   Moderate Pain   Worst Pain

EVENING
0 1 2 3 4 5 6 7 8 9 10
No Pain   Moderate Pain   Worst Pain

WHO ARE YOU MOST THANKFUL FOR?

ANSWER THESE QUESTIONS TO BREAK OUT OF NEGATIVE
THOUGHT PATTERNS AND REFOCUS ON THE THINGS THAT MAKE
YOU HAPPY AND GRATEFUL.

_____
_____
_____
_____
_____
_____
_____
_____
_____
_____

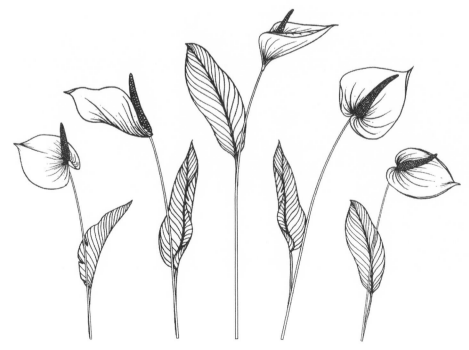

WEEKLY MOOD & PAIN TRACKER - PLOT YOUR MOOD AND PAIN ON THE GRAPH IN DIFFERENT COLORS, KEEP NOTE OF YOUR TRIGGERS BELOW.

PAIN LEVEL

0
1
2
3
4
5
6
7
8
9
10
11
12
13
14
15
16
17

MONDAY	TUESDAY	WEDNESDAY	THURSDAY	FRIDAY	SATURDAY	SUNDAY

TIME OF DAY PAIN TRACKER

MORNING	AFTERNOON	EVENING

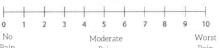

0 1 2 3 4 5 6 7 8 9 10
No Pain   Moderate Pain   Worst Pain

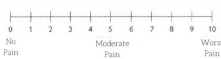

0 1 2 3 4 5 6 7 8 9 10
No Pain   Moderate Pain   Worst Pain

0 1 2 3 4 5 6 7 8 9 10
No Pain   Moderate Pain   Worst Pain

MORNING　　　AFTERNOON　　　EVENING

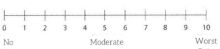

0 1 2 3 4 5 6 7 8 9 10
No Pain   Moderate Pain   Worst Pain

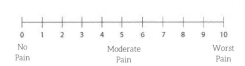

0 1 2 3 4 5 6 7 8 9 10
No Pain   Moderate Pain   Worst Pain

0 1 2 3 4 5 6 7 8 9 10
No Pain   Moderate Pain   Worst Pain

MORNING　　　AFTERNOON　　　EVENING

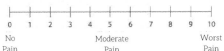

0 1 2 3 4 5 6 7 8 9 10
No Pain   Moderate Pain   Worst Pain

0 1 2 3 4 5 6 7 8 9 10
No Pain   Moderate Pain   Worst Pain

0 1 2 3 4 5 6 7 8 9 10
No Pain   Moderate Pain   Worst Pain

MORNING　　　AFTERNOON　　　EVENING

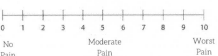

0 1 2 3 4 5 6 7 8 9 10
No Pain   Moderate Pain   Worst Pain

0 1 2 3 4 5 6 7 8 9 10
No Pain   Moderate Pain   Worst Pain

0 1 2 3 4 5 6 7 8 9 10
No Pain   Moderate Pain   Worst Pain

MORNING　　　AFTERNOON　　　EVENING

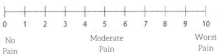

0 1 2 3 4 5 6 7 8 9 10
No Pain   Moderate Pain   Worst Pain

0 1 2 3 4 5 6 7 8 9 10
No Pain   Moderate Pain   Worst Pain

0 1 2 3 4 5 6 7 8 9 10
No Pain   Moderate Pain   Worst Pain

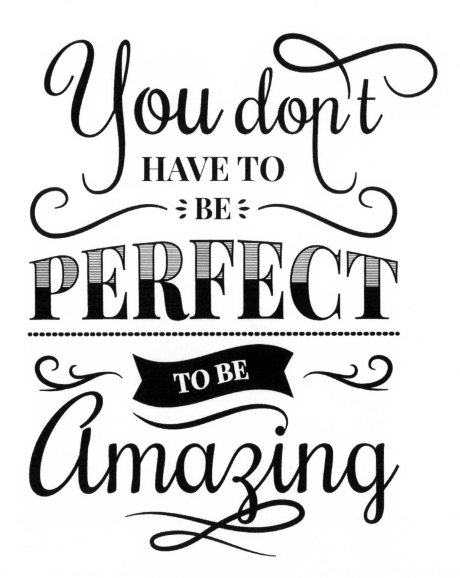

WEEKLY MOOD & PAIN TRACKER - PLOT YOUR MOOD AND PAIN ON THE GRAPH IN DIFFERENT COLORS, KEEP NOTE OF YOUR TRIGGERS BELOW.

PAIN LEVEL

0
1
2
3
4
5
6
7
8
9
10
11
12
13
14
15
16
17

MONDAY   TUESDAY   WEDNESDAY   THURSDAY   FRIDAY   SATURDAY   SUNDAY

TIME OF DAY PAIN TRACKER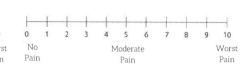

MORNING

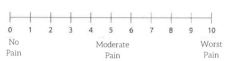

0 1 2 3 4 5 6 7 8 9 10
No Pain   Moderate Pain   Worst Pain

AFTERNOON

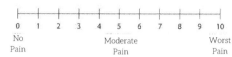

0 1 2 3 4 5 6 7 8 9 10
No Pain   Moderate Pain   Worst Pain

EVENING

0 1 2 3 4 5 6 7 8 9 10
No Pain   Moderate Pain   Worst Pain

MORNING

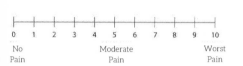

0 1 2 3 4 5 6 7 8 9 10
No Pain   Moderate Pain   Worst Pain

AFTERNOON

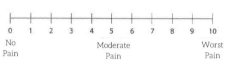

0 1 2 3 4 5 6 7 8 9 10
No Pain   Moderate Pain   Worst Pain

EVENING

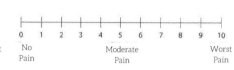

0 1 2 3 4 5 6 7 8 9 10
No Pain   Moderate Pain   Worst Pain

MORNING

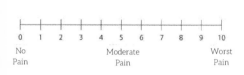

0 1 2 3 4 5 6 7 8 9 10
No Pain   Moderate Pain   Worst Pain

AFTERNOON

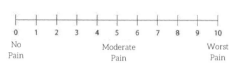

0 1 2 3 4 5 6 7 8 9 10
No Pain   Moderate Pain   Worst Pain

EVENING

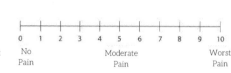

0 1 2 3 4 5 6 7 8 9 10
No Pain   Moderate Pain   Worst Pain

MORNING

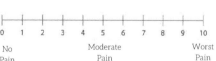
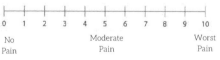

0 1 2 3 4 5 6 7 8 9 10
No Pain   Moderate Pain   Worst Pain

AFTERNOON

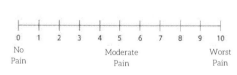

0 1 2 3 4 5 6 7 8 9 10
No Pain   Moderate Pain   Worst Pain

EVENING

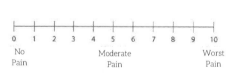

0 1 2 3 4 5 6 7 8 9 10
No Pain   Moderate Pain   Worst Pain

MORNING

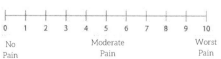

0 1 2 3 4 5 6 7 8 9 10
No Pain   Moderate Pain   Worst Pain

AFTERNOON

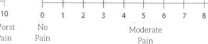

0 1 2 3 4 5 6 7 8 9 10
No Pain   Moderate Pain   Worst Pain

EVENING

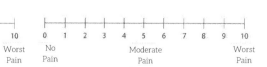

0 1 2 3 4 5 6 7 8 9 10
No Pain   Moderate Pain   Worst Pain

WHAT IS YOUR MOST CHERISHED MEMORY?

ANSWER THESE QUESTIONS TO BREAK OUT OF NEGATIVE
THOUGHT PATTERNS AND REFOCUS ON THE THINGS THAT MAKE
YOU HAPPY AND GRATEFUL.

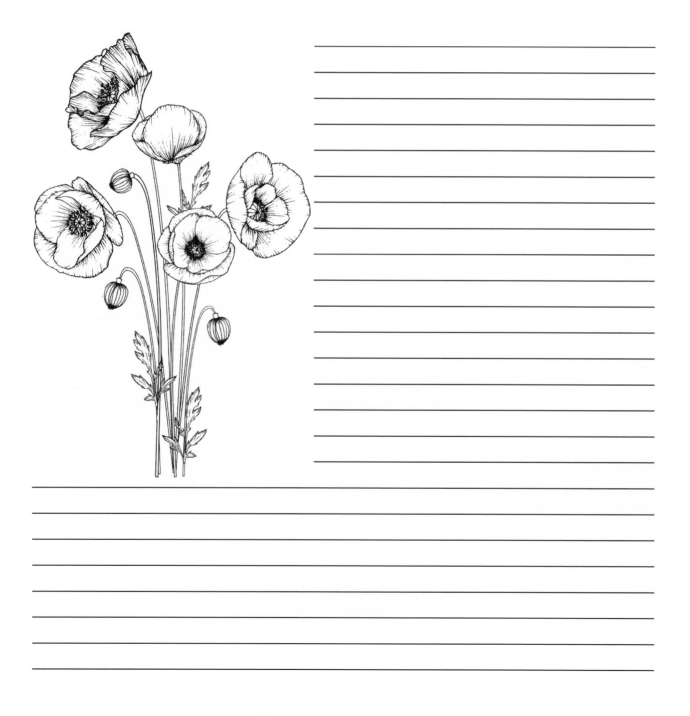

WEEKLY MOOD & PAIN TRACKER - PLOT YOUR MOOD AND PAIN ON THE GRAPH IN DIFFERENT COLORS, KEEP NOTE OF YOUR TRIGGERS BELOW.

PAIN LEVEL

0
1
2
3
4
5
6
7
8
9
10
11
12
13
14
15
16
17

| MONDAY | TUESDAY | WEDNESDAY | THURSDAY | FRIDAY | SATURDAY | SUNDAY |

TIME OF DAY PAIN TRACKER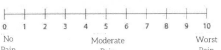

MORNING

0 1 2 3 4 5 6 7 8 9 10
No Pain   Moderate Pain   Worst Pain

AFTERNOON

0 1 2 3 4 5 6 7 8 9 10
No Pain   Moderate Pain   Worst Pain

EVENING

0 1 2 3 4 5 6 7 8 9 10
No Pain   Moderate Pain   Worst Pain

MORNING

0 1 2 3 4 5 6 7 8 9 10
No Pain   Moderate Pain   Worst Pain

AFTERNOON

0 1 2 3 4 5 6 7 8 9 10
No Pain   Moderate Pain   Worst Pain

EVENING

0 1 2 3 4 5 6 7 8 9 10
No Pain   Moderate Pain   Worst Pain

MORNING

0 1 2 3 4 5 6 7 8 9 10
No Pain   Moderate Pain   Worst Pain

AFTERNOON

0 1 2 3 4 5 6 7 8 9 10
No Pain   Moderate Pain   Worst Pain

EVENING

0 1 2 3 4 5 6 7 8 9 10
No Pain   Moderate Pain   Worst Pain

MORNING

0 1 2 3 4 5 6 7 8 9 10
No Pain   Moderate Pain   Worst Pain

AFTERNOON

0 1 2 3 4 5 6 7 8 9 10
No Pain   Moderate Pain   Worst Pain

EVENING

0 1 2 3 4 5 6 7 8 9 10
No Pain   Moderate Pain   Worst Pain

MORNING

0 1 2 3 4 5 6 7 8 9 10
No Pain   Moderate Pain   Worst Pain

AFTERNOON

0 1 2 3 4 5 6 7 8 9 10
No Pain   Moderate Pain   Worst Pain

EVENING

0 1 2 3 4 5 6 7 8 9 10
No Pain   Moderate Pain   Worst Pain

One Minute Meditation

Breathe in through your nose.

Breathe out through your mouth.

Feel air in the depths of your lungs
as you breathe in again.

As you breathe out feel tension
release from your body.

Repeat 3x.

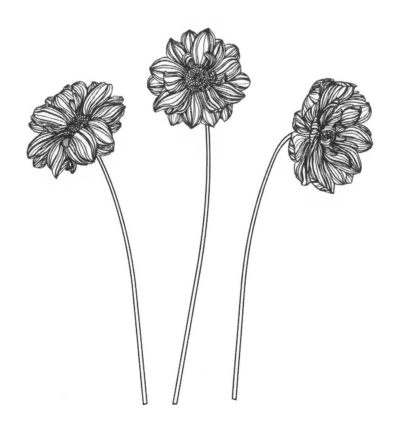

WEEKLY MOOD & PAIN TRACKER - PLOT YOUR MOOD AND PAIN ON THE GRAPH IN DIFFERENT COLORS, KEEP NOTE OF YOUR TRIGGERS BELOW.

PAIN LEVEL

0

1

2

3

4

5

6

7

8

9

10

11

12

13

14

15

16

17

MONDAY	TUESDAY	WEDNESDAY	THURSDAY	FRIDAY	SATURDAY	SUNDAY

TIME OF DAY PAIN TRACKER

MORNING

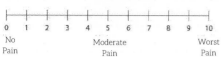

0 1 2 3 4 5 6 7 8 9 10
No Pain   Moderate Pain   Worst Pain

AFTERNOON

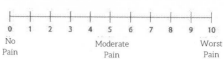

0 1 2 3 4 5 6 7 8 9 10
No Pain   Moderate Pain   Worst Pain

EVENING

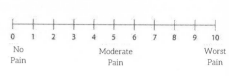

0 1 2 3 4 5 6 7 8 9 10
No Pain   Moderate Pain   Worst Pain

MORNING

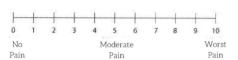

0 1 2 3 4 5 6 7 8 9 10
No Pain   Moderate Pain   Worst Pain

AFTERNOON

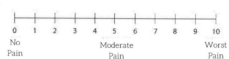

0 1 2 3 4 5 6 7 8 9 10
No Pain   Moderate Pain   Worst Pain

EVENING

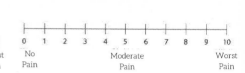

0 1 2 3 4 5 6 7 8 9 10
No Pain   Moderate Pain   Worst Pain

MORNING

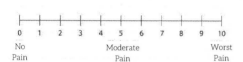

0 1 2 3 4 5 6 7 8 9 10
No Pain   Moderate Pain   Worst Pain

AFTERNOON

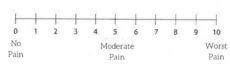

0 1 2 3 4 5 6 7 8 9 10
No Pain   Moderate Pain   Worst Pain

EVENING

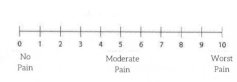

0 1 2 3 4 5 6 7 8 9 10
No Pain   Moderate Pain   Worst Pain

MORNING

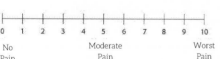
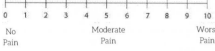

0 1 2 3 4 5 6 7 8 9 10
No Pain   Moderate Pain   Worst Pain

AFTERNOON

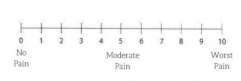

0 1 2 3 4 5 6 7 8 9 10
No Pain   Moderate Pain   Worst Pain

EVENING

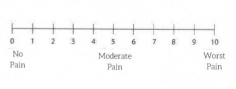

0 1 2 3 4 5 6 7 8 9 10
No Pain   Moderate Pain   Worst Pain

MORNING

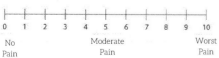
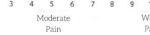

0 1 2 3 4 5 6 7 8 9 10
No Pain   Moderate Pain   Worst Pain

AFTERNOON

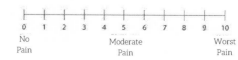

0 1 2 3 4 5 6 7 8 9 10
No Pain   Moderate Pain   Worst Pain

EVENING

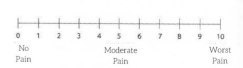

0 1 2 3 4 5 6 7 8 9 10
No Pain   Moderate Pain   Worst Pain

WEEKLY MOOD & PAIN TRACKER - PLOT YOUR MOOD AND PAIN ON THE GRAPH IN DIFFERENT COLORS, KEEP NOTE OF YOUR TRIGGERS BELOW.

PAIN LEVEL

0
1
2
3
4
5
6
7
8
9
10
11
12
13
14
15
16
17

MONDAY	TUESDAY	WEDNESDAY	THURSDAY	FRIDAY	SATURDAY	SUNDAY

TIME OF DAY PAIN TRACKER

MORNING

```
0   1   2   3   4   5   6   7   8   9   10
No                 Moderate              Worst
Pain                 Pain                 Pain
```

AFTERNOON

```
0   1   2   3   4   5   6   7   8   9   10
No                 Moderate              Worst
Pain                 Pain                 Pain
```

EVENING

```
0   1   2   3   4   5   6   7   8   9   10
No                 Moderate              Worst
Pain                 Pain                 Pain
```

MORNING

```
0   1   2   3   4   5   6   7   8   9   10
No                 Moderate              Worst
Pain                 Pain                 Pain
```

AFTERNOON

```
0   1   2   3   4   5   6   7   8   9   10
No                 Moderate              Worst
Pain                 Pain                 Pain
```

EVENING

```
0   1   2   3   4   5   6   7   8   9   10
No                 Moderate              Worst
Pain                 Pain                 Pain
```

MORNING

```
0   1   2   3   4   5   6   7   8   9   10
No                 Moderate              Worst
Pain                 Pain                 Pain
```

AFTERNOON

```
0   1   2   3   4   5   6   7   8   9   10
No                 Moderate              Worst
Pain                 Pain                 Pain
```

EVENING

```
0   1   2   3   4   5   6   7   8   9   10
No                 Moderate              Worst
Pain                 Pain                 Pain
```

MORNING

```
0   1   2   3   4   5   6   7   8   9   10
No                 Moderate              Worst
Pain                 Pain                 Pain
```

AFTERNOON

```
0   1   2   3   4   5   6   7   8   9   10
No                 Moderate              Worst
Pain                 Pain                 Pain
```

EVENING

```
0   1   2   3   4   5   6   7   8   9   10
No                 Moderate              Worst
Pain                 Pain                 Pain
```

MORNING

```
0   1   2   3   4   5   6   7   8   9   10
No                 Moderate              Worst
Pain                 Pain                 Pain
```

AFTERNOON

```
0   1   2   3   4   5   6   7   8   9   10
No                 Moderate              Worst
Pain                 Pain                 Pain
```

EVENING

```
0   1   2   3   4   5   6   7   8   9   10
No                 Moderate              Worst
Pain                 Pain                 Pain
```

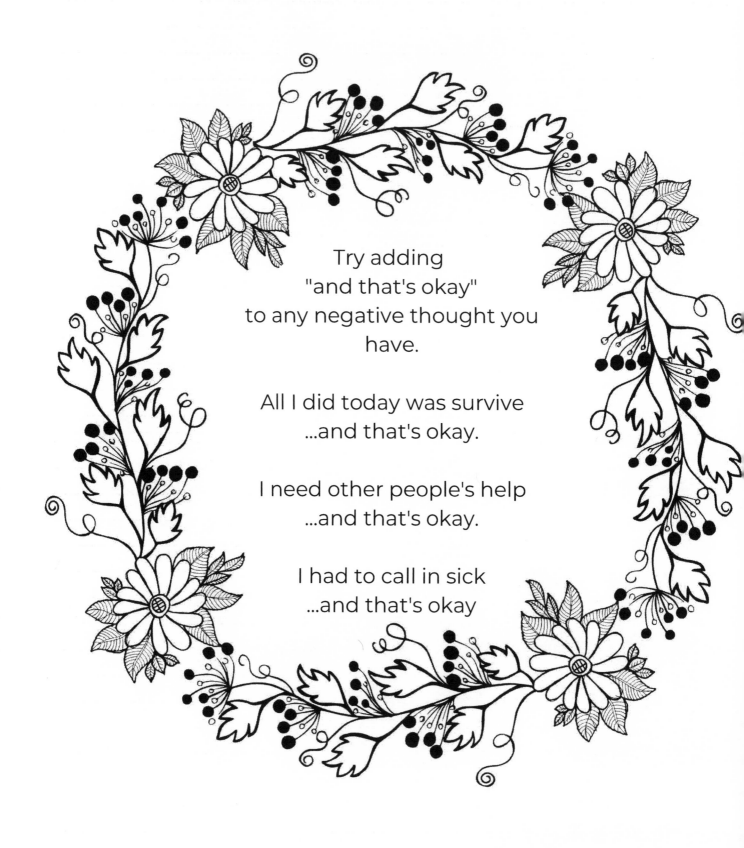

Try adding
"and that's okay"
to any negative thought you
have.

All I did today was survive
...and that's okay.

I need other people's help
...and that's okay.

I had to call in sick
...and that's okay

WEEKLY MOOD & PAIN TRACKER - PLOT YOUR MOOD AND PAIN ON THE GRAPH IN DIFFERENT COLORS, KEEP NOTE OF YOUR TRIGGERS BELOW.

PAIN LEVEL

0
1
2
3
4
5
6
7
8
9
10
11
12
13
14
15
16
17

MONDAY	TUESDAY	WEDNESDAY	THURSDAY	FRIDAY	SATURDAY	SUNDAY

TIME OF DAY PAIN TRACKER

MORNING

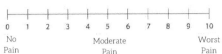

No Pain   Moderate Pain   Worst Pain

AFTERNOON

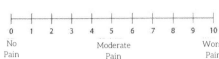

No Pain   Moderate Pain   Worst Pain

EVENING

No Pain   Moderate Pain   Worst Pain

MORNING

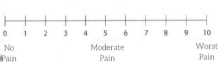

No Pain   Moderate Pain   Worst Pain

AFTERNOON

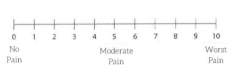

No Pain   Moderate Pain   Worst Pain

EVENING

No Pain   Moderate Pain   Worst Pain

MORNING

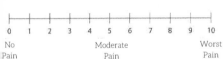

No Pain   Moderate Pain   Worst Pain

AFTERNOON

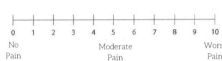

No Pain   Moderate Pain   Worst Pain

EVENING

No Pain   Moderate Pain   Worst Pain

MORNING

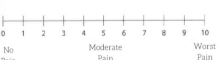

No Pain   Moderate Pain   Worst Pain

AFTERNOON

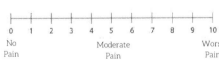

No Pain   Moderate Pain   Worst Pain

EVENING

No Pain   Moderate Pain   Worst Pain

MORNING

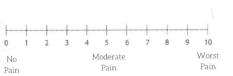

No Pain   Moderate Pain   Worst Pain

AFTERNOON

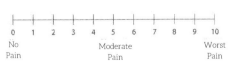

No Pain   Moderate Pain   Worst Pain

EVENING

No Pain   Moderate Pain   Worst Pain

WEEKLY MOOD & PAIN TRACKER - PLOT YOUR MOOD AND PAIN ON THE GRAPH IN DIFFERENT COLORS, KEEP NOTE OF YOUR TRIGGERS BELOW.

PAIN LEVEL

0
1
2
3
4
5
6
7
8
9
10
11
12
13
14
15
16
17

MONDAY	TUESDAY	WEDNESDAY	THURSDAY	FRIDAY	SATURDAY	SUNDAY

TIME OF DAY PAIN TRACKER

MORNING

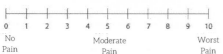

0 1 2 3 4 5 6 7 8 9 10
No Pain   Moderate Pain   Worst Pain

AFTERNOON

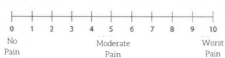

0 1 2 3 4 5 6 7 8 9 10
No Pain   Moderate Pain   Worst Pain

EVENING

0 1 2 3 4 5 6 7 8 9 10
No Pain   Moderate Pain   Worst Pain

MORNING

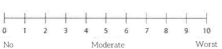

0 1 2 3 4 5 6 7 8 9 10
No Pain   Moderate Pain   Worst Pain

AFTERNOON

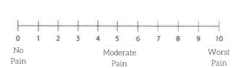

0 1 2 3 4 5 6 7 8 9 10
No Pain   Moderate Pain   Worst Pain

EVENING

0 1 2 3 4 5 6 7 8 9 10
No Pain   Moderate Pain   Worst Pain

MORNING

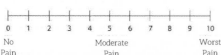

0 1 2 3 4 5 6 7 8 9 10
No Pain   Moderate Pain   Worst Pain

AFTERNOON

0 1 2 3 4 5 6 7 8 9 10
No Pain   Moderate Pain   Worst Pain

EVENING

0 1 2 3 4 5 6 7 8 9 10
No Pain   Moderate Pain   Worst Pain

MORNING

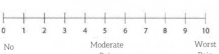

0 1 2 3 4 5 6 7 8 9 10
No Pain   Moderate Pain   Worst Pain

AFTERNOON

0 1 2 3 4 5 6 7 8 9 10
No Pain   Moderate Pain   Worst Pain

EVENING

0 1 2 3 4 5 6 7 8 9 10
No Pain   Moderate Pain   Worst Pain

MORNING

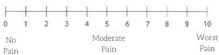

0 1 2 3 4 5 6 7 8 9 10
No Pain   Moderate Pain   Worst Pain

AFTERNOON

0 1 2 3 4 5 6 7 8 9 10
No Pain   Moderate Pain   Worst Pain

EVENING

0 1 2 3 4 5 6 7 8 9 10
No Pain   Moderate Pain   Worst Pain

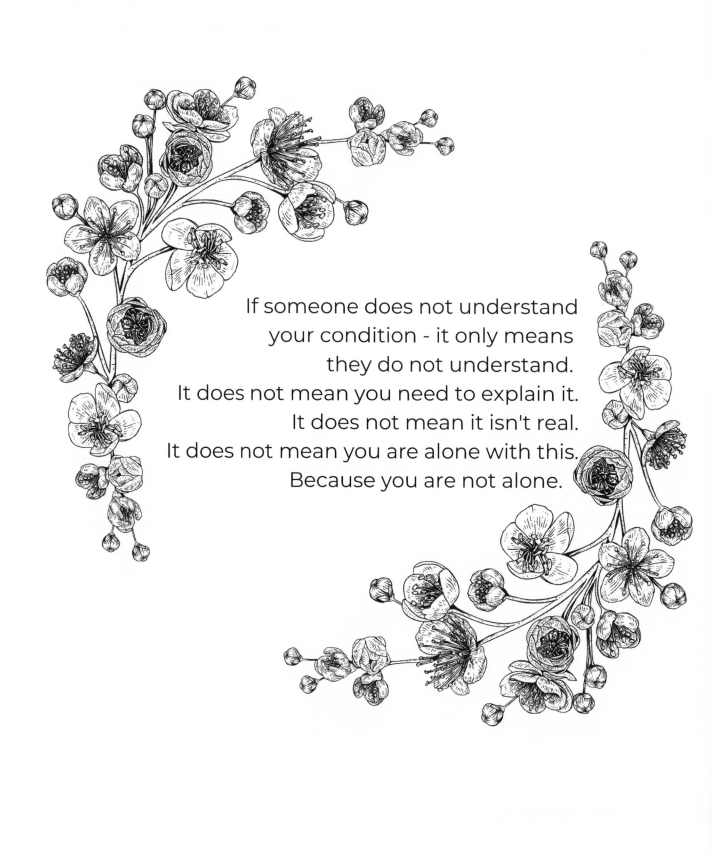

If someone does not understand
your condition - it only means
they do not understand.
It does not mean you need to explain it.
It does not mean it isn't real.
It does not mean you are alone with this.
Because you are not alone.

WEEKLY MOOD & PAIN TRACKER - PLOT YOUR MOOD AND PAIN ON THE GRAPH IN DIFFERENT COLORS, KEEP NOTE OF YOUR TRIGGERS BELOW.

PAIN LEVEL

0

1

2

3

4

5

6

7

8

9

10

11

12

13

14

15

16

17

MONDAY	TUESDAY	WEDNESDAY	THURSDAY	FRIDAY	SATURDAY	SUNDAY

TIME OF DAY PAIN TRACKER

MORNING

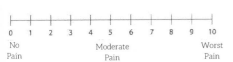

0 1 2 3 4 5 6 7 8 9 10

No Pain   Moderate Pain   Worst Pain

AFTERNOON

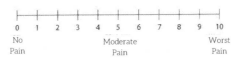

0 1 2 3 4 5 6 7 8 9 10

No Pain   Moderate Pain   Worst Pain

EVENING

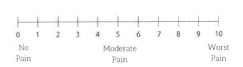

0 1 2 3 4 5 6 7 8 9 10

No Pain   Moderate Pain   Worst Pain

MORNING

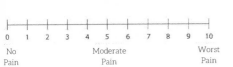

0 1 2 3 4 5 6 7 8 9 10

No Pain   Moderate Pain   Worst Pain

AFTERNOON

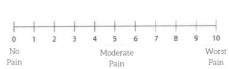

0 1 2 3 4 5 6 7 8 9 10

No Pain   Moderate Pain   Worst Pain

EVENING

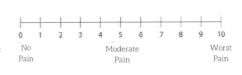

0 1 2 3 4 5 6 7 8 9 10

No Pain   Moderate Pain   Worst Pain

MORNING

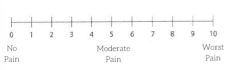

0 1 2 3 4 5 6 7 8 9 10

No Pain   Moderate Pain   Worst Pain

AFTERNOON

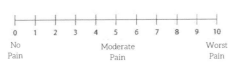

0 1 2 3 4 5 6 7 8 9 10

No Pain   Moderate Pain   Worst Pain

EVENING

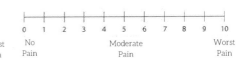

0 1 2 3 4 5 6 7 8 9 10

No Pain   Moderate Pain   Worst Pain

MORNING

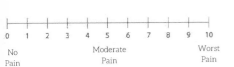

0 1 2 3 4 5 6 7 8 9 10

No Pain   Moderate Pain   Worst Pain

AFTERNOON

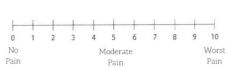

0 1 2 3 4 5 6 7 8 9 10

No Pain   Moderate Pain   Worst Pain

EVENING

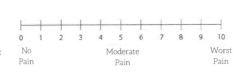

0 1 2 3 4 5 6 7 8 9 10

No Pain   Moderate Pain   Worst Pain

MORNING

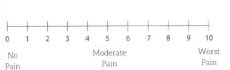

0 1 2 3 4 5 6 7 8 9 10

No Pain   Moderate Pain   Worst Pain

AFTERNOON

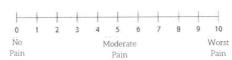

0 1 2 3 4 5 6 7 8 9 10

No Pain   Moderate Pain   Worst Pain

EVENING

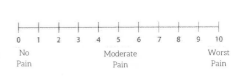

0 1 2 3 4 5 6 7 8 9 10

No Pain   Moderate Pain   Worst Pain

WHAT BODY PART ARE YOU GRATEFUL FOR?

ANSWER THESE QUESTIONS TO BREAK OUT OF NEGATIVE
THOUGHT PATTERNS AND REFOCUS ON THE THINGS THAT MAKE
YOU HAPPY AND GRATEFUL.

Made in the USA
Middletown, DE
21 February 2019